PHILIPPA FAULKS

GATEWAYS TO HEALTH

SECRETS OF MEDITATION

SIMPLE TECHNIQUES FOR ACHIEVING HARMONY

WATKINS PUBLISHING
LONDON

Distributed in the USA and Canada by
Sterling Publishing Co., Inc.
387 Park Avenue South, New York, NY 10016

This edition published in the UK 2009 by
Watkins Publishing, Sixth Floor, Castle House,
75–76 Wells Street, London W1T 3QH

Conceived, created and designed by Duncan Baird Publishers

1 3 5 7 9 10 8 6 4 2

Designed by Clare Thorpe
Commissioned artwork by Art-4

Printed and bound in Great Britain

Library of Congress Cataloging-in-Publication Data Available

ISBN: 978-1-906787-04-2

www.watkinspublishing.co.uk

For information about custom editions, special sales, premium
and corporate purchases, please contact Sterling Special Sales
Department at 800-805-5489 or specialsales@sterlingpub.com

Contents

Introduction

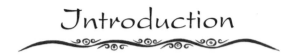

From its ancient beginnings, the art of meditation has developed into a structured practice over thousands of years and is used today by millions of people worldwide. It is truly universal, and is incorporated into the doctrines and practices of differing nationalities and religious beliefs. The best-known spiritual paths include:

Hinduism (India) Indian scriptures dating back 5000 years describe meditation techniques. Hinduism traditionally has six schools of yoga incorporating meditation as a core practice.

Buddhism (India/China/Japan/Tibet) Meditation is central to all forms of Buddhism.

Christianity The use of prayer, the rosary and the Adoration are all forms of meditation.

Judaism Jewish meditation dates back thousands of years. There are two Old Testament words for meditation — *hagâ* (to meditate) and *sîhâ* (to muse/ rehearse in one's mind).

Islam Mohammed spent long periods in meditation and this practice is fundamental to the mystical side of Islam (Sufism).

Many other faiths record or depict the practice of meditation. To give an example, in Ancient Egypt the spiritual practice of the temple priests involved many hours of meditation. Pharaoh is traditionally shown seated in the 'Throne posture' – a position often used for deep meditation.

Taoism, Krishnamurti and Osho, are further examples of faiths which have espoused the benefits and wisdom of meditation, often with a very different concept.

Taoism (Daoism) uses 'meditation in motion' in the form of Tai Chi.

Krishnamurti believed that we should remove choice and the need to strive; meditation to him was about choiceless awareness in the present moment.

Osho (formerly *Rajneesh*) created 'Active/Dynamic Meditation', where the person is in a state of movement followed by silence.

What is Meditation?

Meditation is the practice of focusing on an object, thought or sound, often of a singular nature. The purpose is to calm and clear the mind, so creating a peaceful state whereby we can achieve deep relaxation or a more spiritual state of awareness.

Our minds are often full of a variety of thoughts, good and bad, which can become overwhelming in everyday life. Meditation allows us to stop and unravel those thoughts, giving us a short period in time where all is still, and either our focus is on one fixed thing or our mind is devoid of all thought. This can have a similar effect on our brain as defragmenting our computer – shifting all our thoughts into the correct filing system and allowing us to think more clearly and be more aware of our mind and emotions, giving us the chance to achieve equilibrium.

Health Benefits of Meditation

Meditation does not have to be a religious or spiritual practice. Many secular groups practise meditation for the positive mental and physical benefits — Progressive Muscle Relaxation, the Relaxation Response and Biofeedback all use techniques drawn from the various spiritual practices but without the doctrine.

Recent medical clinical studies have found that meditation can have a positive effect on stress-related illness, immune function, chronic or terminal illness, cardiovascular and respiratory functions (high blood pressure/heart problems etc), and brain chemistry.

More and more data is becoming available to show the progressive benefits of meditation with or without a spiritual concept and it is now being offered by the Health Service to patients in the UK for stress and pain reduction.

When Should I Meditate?

There are no hard and fast rules as to when you should meditate, but to get a real benefit from meditating, it is advisable to dedicate at least one twenty-minute slot every day when you know you will not be disturbed — make time for yourself by unplugging/switching off all phones and devices, and asking any family or friends who are around not to disturb you. Once you make the commitment to meditate, you will find a time to suit your daily routine. You may also like to use a timer that can rouse you at the end of your twenty minutes.

Try to build up to *two* twenty-minute sessions a day for optimum benefit.

If you are travelling you may have to adapt your time slots but when you are more experienced you can make use of the time on the train or plane to 'disconnect' from daily life.

Where Should I Meditate?

Again this is entirely up to you but initially it needs to be somewhere quiet, comfortable and free from distraction. Do not attempt to meditate in a cluttered, noisy environment — try to keep your meditation area as calm and minimal as possible.

We will discuss shortly how you should sit but you may wish to have a choice of a chair, cushions, a blanket, etc.

Keep the room comfortably warm or cool depending on the weather and you can add little touches such as incense, a statue or natural objects to your meditation area as you wish. In time, when you are an experienced 'meditator' you may find you are able to meditate almost anywhere — outside, on a train or even in a thunder storm — without becoming uncomfortable or distracted.

How to Practise

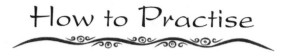

Relaxation & Beginning

Before you begin to meditate properly, it is often useful to learn how to relax. This may sound ridiculous but in the modern world we have almost forgotten how to be completely at ease in our body. Often we have a nagging ache or area of tension and if you are going to be sitting or lying in one position, it is important that you are comfortable. When you have learnt this simple relaxation technique, you will find it easy to lie or sit and calm yourself quickly and with ease.

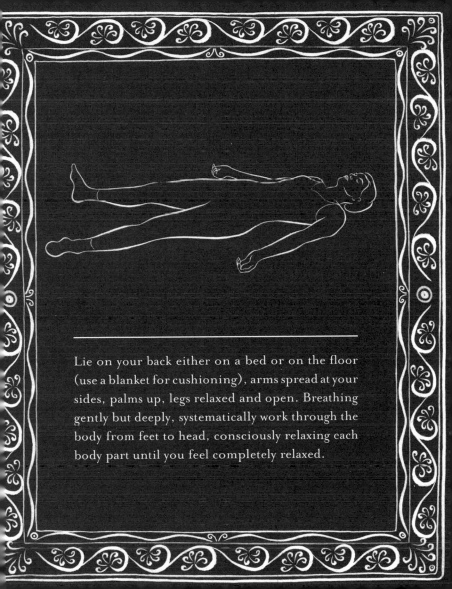

Lie on your back either on a bed or on the floor (use a blanket for cushioning), arms spread at your sides, palms up, legs relaxed and open. Breathing gently but deeply, systematically work through the body from feet to head, consciously relaxing each body part until you feel completely relaxed.

Sitting Postures

Burmese

This is one of the simplest and most comfortable postures to start with for meditation.

In the Burmese posture the legs are not crossed, the knees are turned outwards to the floor. The legs are bent and the feet placed in front of the pelvis with one foot in front of the other. Your hands rest on the knees, at the top of the thighs or on the heels. Feel free to adjust the position of the feet until you are comfortable; it is perfectly acceptable either to have the feet straight in front of each other or to let them pass so that one foot is next to the other ankle. You may have to adjust the angle slightly to allow you to place your calves or knees on the floor.

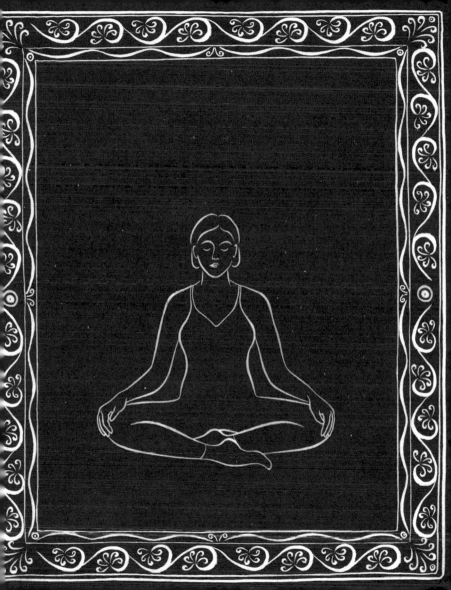

Half and Full Lotus

These sitting positions are the ones most commonly associated with meditation; however, they are not the easiest to begin with. Please do not attempt to achieve these postures without first doing a proper course in yoga or stretching.

Half Lotus

1 Sitting cross-legged, place the outside foot on the inner thigh, sole facing upward, with the hands in the *gyan* position on your knees (see page 22).

Full Lotus

2 Sitting cross-legged, place both feet, soles upwards on opposite thighs, with the hands in *gyan*.

If sitting cross-legged does not suit you find another position that does – meditation should be comfortable.

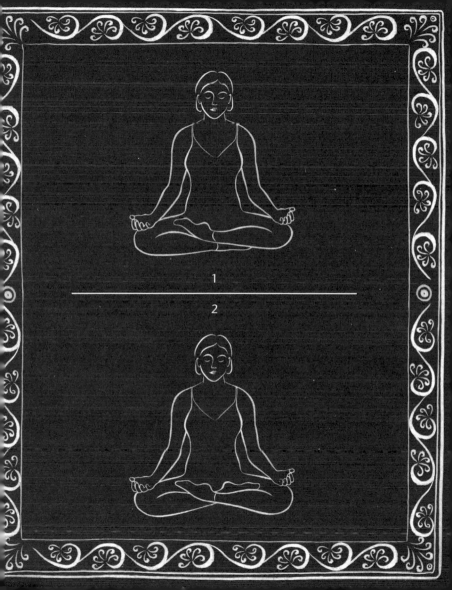

Throne Posture

Throne posture is excellent if you are unable to sit cross-legged or in a kneeling posture. You will need a straight-backed chair, where you can sit comfortably with your feet placed flat on the floor and your back supported as pictured. Relax the shoulders down without slouching and rest the hands gently on your thighs. Try and keep the chin slightly raised and the spine erect.

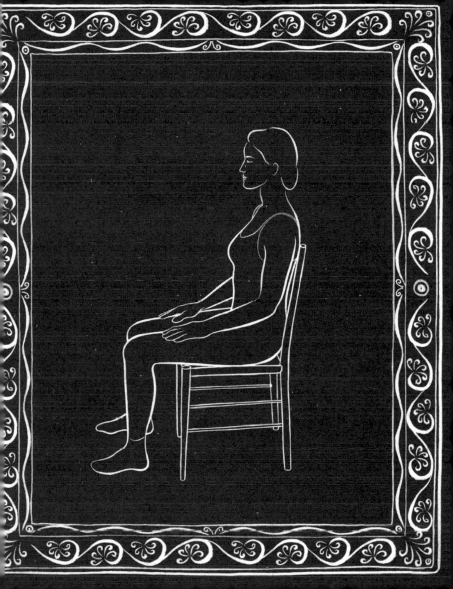

Kneeling Posture

Kneeling is another useful position if you can't sit cross-legged. There are special meditation "kneeling benches" you can purchase to make it more comfortable but you can also place a cushion between your buttocks and your feet. Experiment with your position until you find it most comfortable. Do not feel restricted to any one posture, in fact some meditations occasionally require a different position to the one you may be used to.

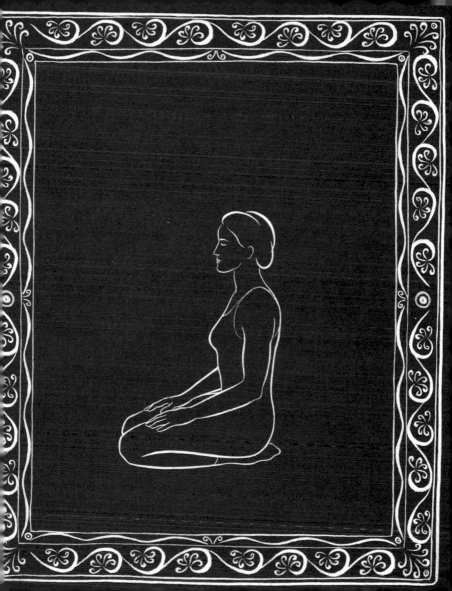

Breathing Techniques

The importance of good breathing during meditation is two-fold. Not only does it allow you to use the breath as a focus and aid to relaxation, it also feeds the body with oxygen. Most of us only use a third of our lung capacity and deep, gentle breathing allows us to fill our lungs more efficiently, which in turn gives us the vital oxygen our organs and blood need to keep our cells healthy and our brain focused and alert. Use the deep breathing technique on its own at intervals during the day to calm and focus yourself.

Your breathing should be slow, deep and gentle. Breathe in through the nose filling the abdomen rather than the chest. Your abdomen should slowly inflate on the in-breath and deflate on the out-breath. Then gently release the air back through your mouth.

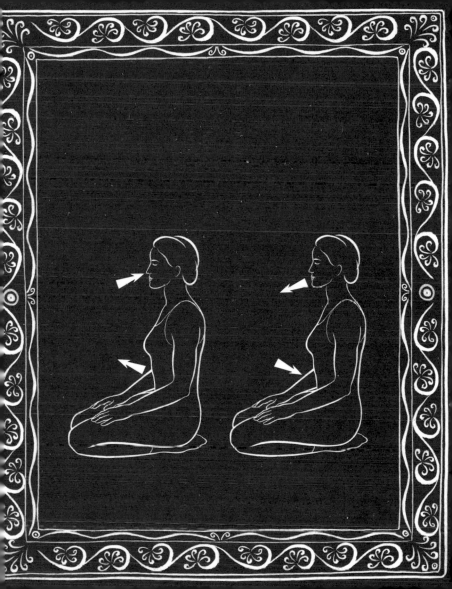

Mudras
(Hand Positions)

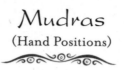

Mudra means 'seal' in Sanskrit and is a symbolic or ritual gesture mainly used in Hinduism or Buddhism. They are primarily made using the hands and each position is believed to have a specific effect. They are used in traditional Indian dance but also for the practice of meditation.

Gyan

1 This position symbolizes the 'starting point' and helps clear the mind and grounds the body. The thumb and index finger touch and the other fingers relax in a curve as shown; rest the hands on the thighs.

Dhyana

2 *Dhyana* is another very simple but calming hand position, also known as the 'meditation pose'. Rest the left hand palm up in the palm of the right hand with your thumbs touching.

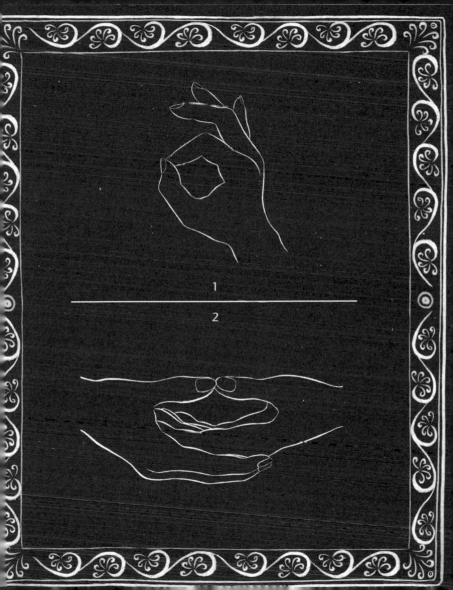

Akash

3   If you wish to 'centre' yourself, *Akash* mudra can help nourish the parts of your body that are lacking in energy. Join the thumb and middle finger, whilst extending the remaining fingers.

Vajra

4   *Vajra* (5 Element Fist) mudra helps transform ignorance to wisdom — it brings into balance the five elements of earth, air, fire, water and metal. The right hand encloses the left index finger in a fist, the thumb placed over the tip of the finger. The left hand can make a fist below the right.

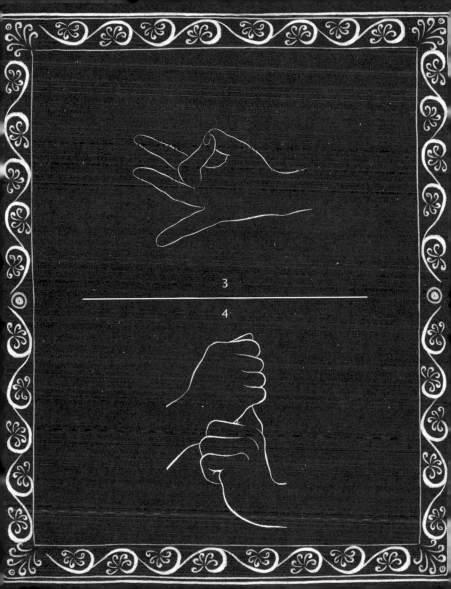

3

4

Uttarabodhi

5   *Uttarabodhi* mudra symbolizes perfection and is associated with supreme power/divine providence. The hands are clasped together in the lap, index fingers extended and touching, the rest of the fingers crossed and folded down.

Mida-no Jouin

6   *Mida-no Jouin* mudra represents duality and the two worlds, the hands mirroring each other. The hands rest in the lap, the last three fingers interlaced to create an overlapping platform. The index fingers form two upward circles, the tips touching the thumbs.

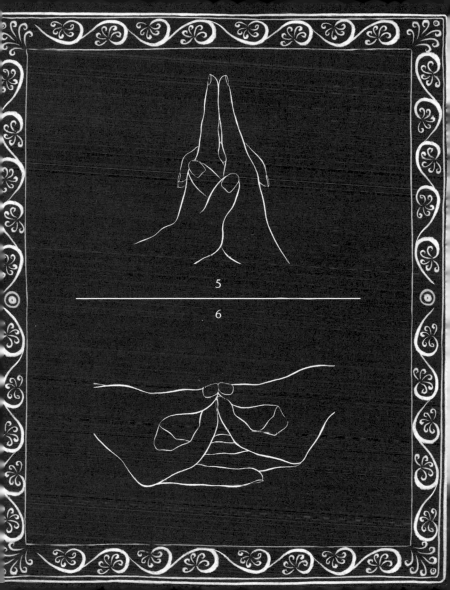

5

6

Mandalas for Meditation

Mandala means 'circle' or 'completion' in Sanskrit. It is modernly a generic term that refers to various objects, plans, charts or geometric patterns that can be created and contemplated upon. These patterns represent the Universe from a microcosmic (the smallest) point of view.

In the various spiritual traditions mentioned previously, Mandalas are used to create a 'sacred place' and to aid meditation by creating a sense of 'oneness' or 'unity' with the forces of the universe.

Unity Mandala

The ancient cross within the circle. The circle represents eternity and the cross is the juxtaposition between the material and the divine. Focus on this symbol to achieve humanity, spiritual and material balance.

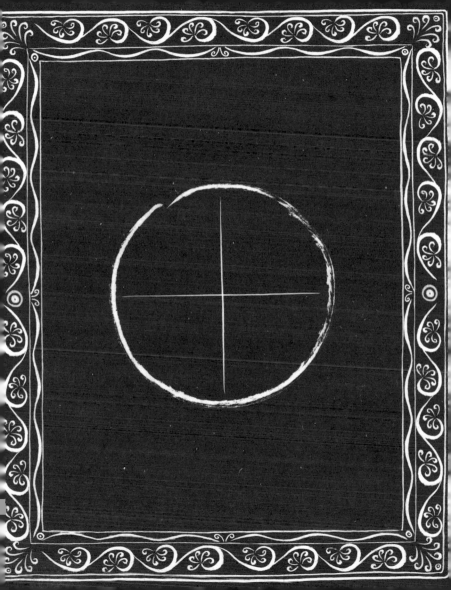

Lotus Mandala

The lotus flower is used in many spiritual traditions as a symbol of purity and eternity. The lotus flower grows in mud but remains untouched by it, thus symbolizing our ability to transcend the material world and become divine, untainted by the base elements of human nature. The ancients were also transfixed by the way the lotus opens its petals at sunrise and closes them at sunset — to them this represented the endless cycle of life, death and rebirth.

Meditate upon the lotus to help triumph over negative or base emotions and to find joy in the cycle of life.

Chakra Mandala

Chakras are the energy centres within the body, represented by circles of colour. They correspond to the nerve centres and organs in the body. The Chakra Mandala can be used to focus on these areas to balance the energy and facilitate healing.

Base Chakra (red) — bottom of spine — adrenals, elimination process — primal life force
Sacral Chakra (orange) — genitals — reproductive organs — emotion, sexual energy
Solar Plexus (yellow) — navel — digestive organs — self-will, identity, mental processes
Heart Chakra (green) — heart — respiratory organs — love, compassion, healing
Throat Chakra (blue) — laryngeal pluxus — thyroid — self-expression, speech
Third Eye Chakra (indigo) — between brows — pituitary — intuition, psychism
Crown Chakra (violet) — top of head — pineal gland — peace, divinity, enlightenment

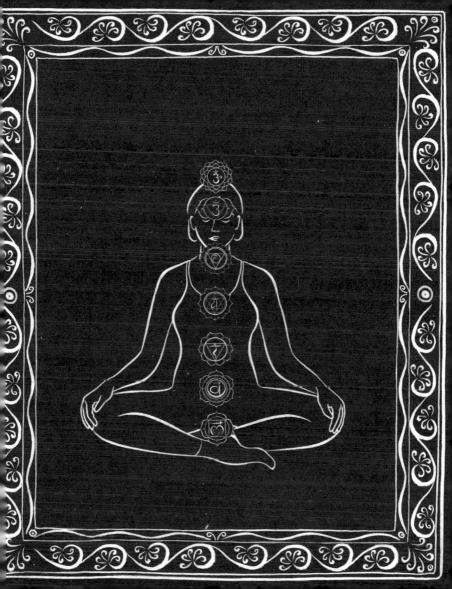

Elemental Mandala

The four elements — earth, air, fire and water — have been universally used throughout history. The ancient Greek philosophers believed that these four elements were the root of all matter. The fifth element is 'Spirit' and completes the cycle.

Twentieth-century healer and magician Franz Bardon wrote that the positive and negative traits of the elements could affect the human body, mind and spirit. Through conscious positive contemplation and balancing, elemental harmony can be achieved.

Earth (black/brown/green) — material, grounding, finances
Air (yellow) — intellect, communication
Fire (red) — self-will, power, passions, creativity, sexuality
Water (blue) — emotions, relationships
Spirit (white/purple) — spirituality, divine communion

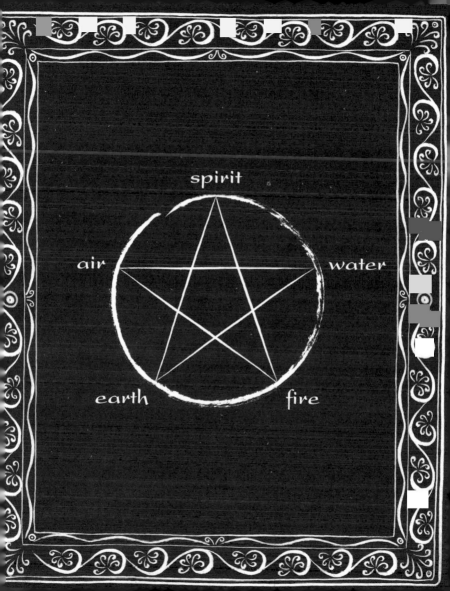

Seed of Life Mandala

The 'Seed of Life' is a symbol of the seven days of creation and is a perfect example of Sacred Geometry. One of the earliest depictions is on the wall of an ancient Egyptian temple at Abydos.

If you unravel the pattern you can see the steps of Creation, beginning with the first circle. If you add to the pattern, the Seed becomes a Flower and then a Fruit which contains the blueprint of the Universe.

This Mandala can be used for contemplation on the process of creation, not only of the Universe but of ourselves. It is also traditionally a symbol of blessing, protection and fertility.

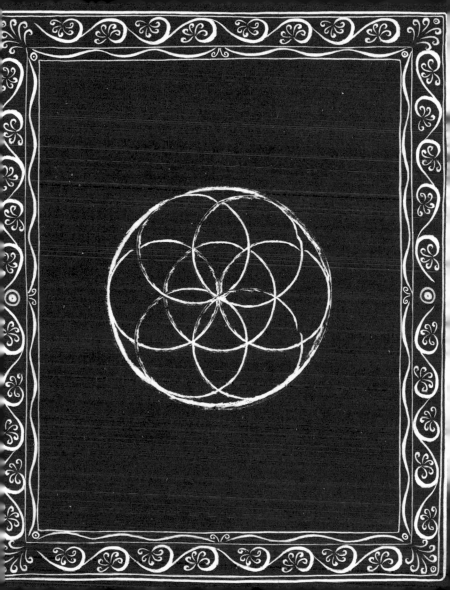

Mantras

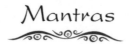

A mantra is a word, phrase, sound or vibration used in repetition. It is used to create a one-point of concentration or even as a spiritual communication. A commonly recognized mantra is the Buddhist 'OM' or even the use of the Rosary (the Catholic prayer consisting of the Lord's Prayer, Hail Mary, etc).

Mantras can be used alongside meditation as a deeply spiritual exercise or on a more subtle level as a method of auto-suggestion. Both can create a deep sense of calmness.

A simple mantra would be to use and focus on the word 'Calm' during your meditation. Breathe in, silently say 'Calm', and gently release the breath. Repeat as long as you wish, focusing totally on the word, maybe even visualizing the letters as if written in your mind.

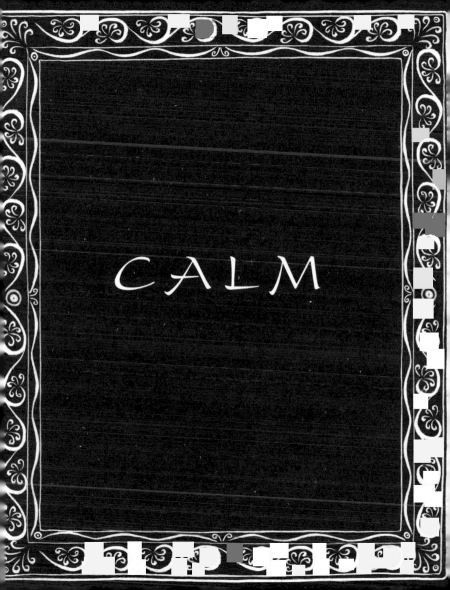

CALM

Mantras with Beads

One simple way of helping to keep your mind on your point of focus when meditating with mantras is to use a string of beads. This is an ancient technique and one we recognize easily from the use of the prayer beads of the Rosary (the string of beads with a crucifix as used by Catholics). The beads allow us to mentally 'keep count' of our mantra and so let the mind concentrate on the meditation process. The usual amount of beads used for meditation is 108 but it is not totally necessary to have this exact number.

You can use any type of beaded string – wooden, gemstone, glass or even plastic – and they can be fixed or moveable along the string, whichever you find most comfortable.

As you say your 'word/mantra', move or pass your fingers over one bead at a time and then repeat until the end of the string.

Meditations

Emerging Lotus Meditation

Lotus Light Meditation

Protection Meditation

Stop-the-Clock Meditation

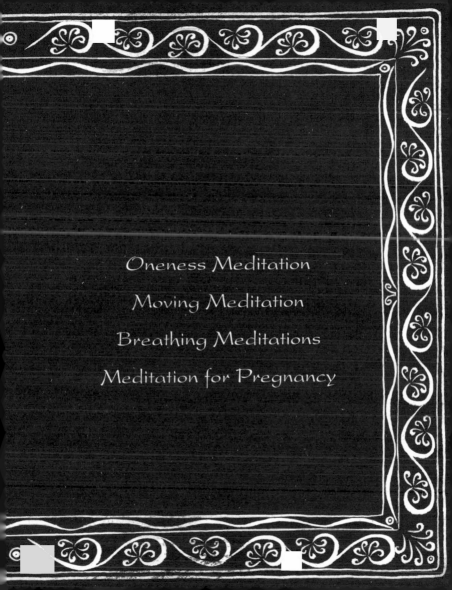

Oneness Meditation

Moving Meditation

Breathing Meditations

Meditation for Pregnancy

Emerging Lotus Meditation

Sit in whichever posture you are comfortable with. Begin to breathe gently and slowly and as you do so focus on a feeling of being enveloped in a comforting darkness. Continue to focus on your breath and gradually sense that you are surrounded by the petals of a lotus flower, tightly budded. Breathe and focus on being enveloped in darkness. Slowly begin to feel the petals unfurl, one by one. Each petal can represent a part of your self that is opening up to the world or to spirit. Breathe and focus, see the light begin to creep in as each petal unfolds. When all the petals have unfurled, you are seated within the lotus flower surrounded and bathed in the bright light of the sun. Breathe in the light and know that you are reborn.

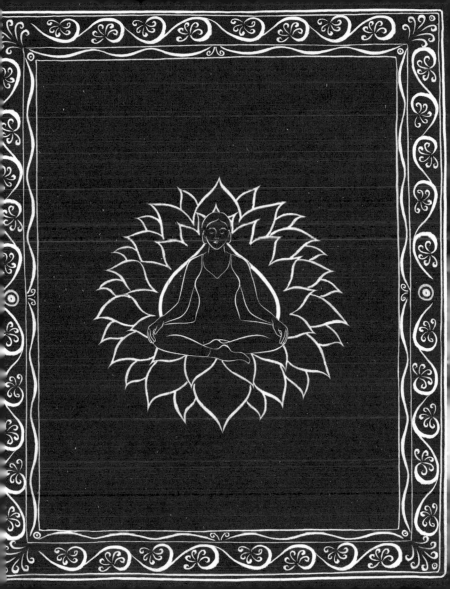

Lotus Light Meditation

Sit in your comfortable position and as you breathe in, imagine that with every breath you breathe in a glowing white light. Focus the light into one small glowing point in your *Dantien* (the centre of your body three finger-widths below your navel). With each breath this tiny bead of light grows. Imagine that it radiates health and harmony as it shines and as you do so imagine it growing in size, forming into the bud of a lotus flower. When the time is right, the lotus bud will start to open inside you. The petals divide into shards of light and soon your whole torso will contain this flower. When this happens a great calmness ensues. Keep your mind on this image for the remainder of the meditation, knowing that balance, health and harmony are within you.

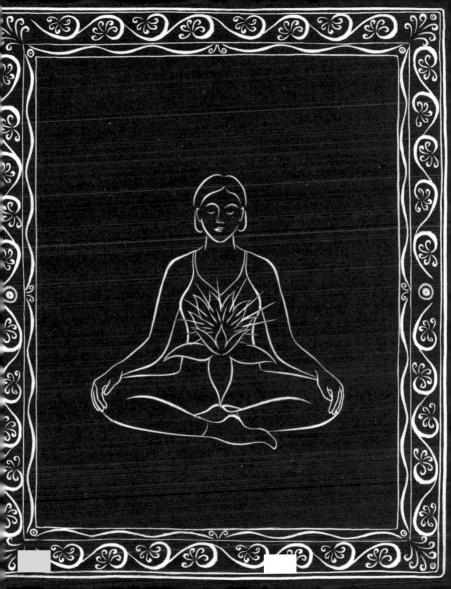

Protection Meditation

Sit in your preferred posture, hands resting on your knees or thighs. Breathe gently and focus on the breath, gradually imagining and building up a sphere of light around you. The light may be pure white or whatever colour you find comfortable, soothing or protective. Focus on your breath and reinforce the sphere of light, making it brighter and more solid as you concentrate on the regular in and out movement of your breath. Continue this until you feel that the sphere is completely enveloping your entire being and that it contains only pure and positive light. Hold this feeling until you are ready to absorb the light into yourself and do so by breathing in deeply. Hold the breath for a second or two and then exhale, holding onto the absorbed light.

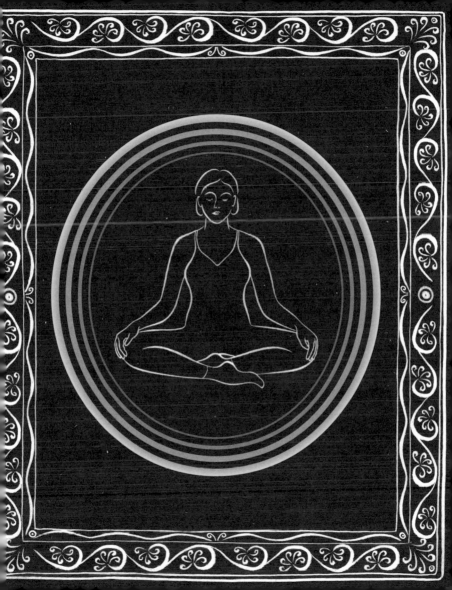

Stop-the-Clock Meditation

This meditation focuses on stillness, the art of being totally in the present, what is traditionally called 'Mindfulness Meditation'. Mindfulness is being aware of your thoughts, actions or motivations and it is now known to have a very beneficial effect on many stress-related disorders. The object of mindfulness is to experience what is happening in the 'now' and deal with the sensation or thought carefully and rationally.

Sit comfortably. Breathe regularly and deeply, allowing all thoughts to pass by without reaction. You are firmly in the present focusing on each breath. Do not examine anything, merely acknowledge and allow it to pass. Any image, thought or distraction is irrelevant; continue to focus solely on your breathing, on being totally in the present moment. With continued practice this meditation can create patience, acceptance and peace.

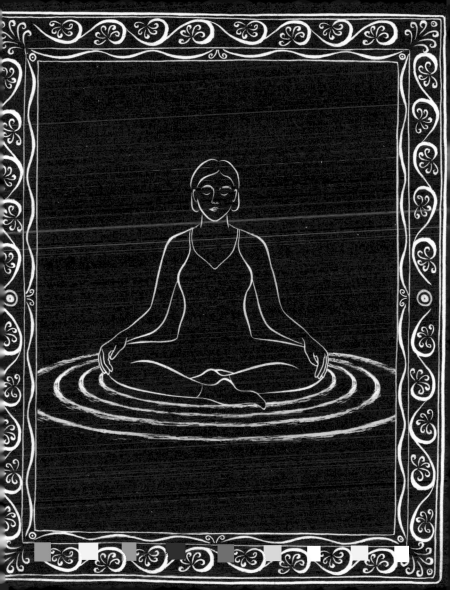

Oneness Meditation

This meditation helps reconnect us to the 'source', the very beginning of our creation or destiny.

Sit comfortably and take a breath in. Hold the breath for a few heartbeats so that you become fully aware of 'you'. Continue breathing rhythmically and gently, becoming more aware of the relativity of your self, the room, the outside world and gradually the universe around you. Experience the depth and vastness as you concentrate on your breath and your 'being'. If you are religious, reach out with each breath to your God; begin to feel that deep connection with the very being that created you. If you have no religious path, extend yourself to whatever 'essence' or 'being' you feel you evolved from. When you feel the connection, with each breath extend it to every living thing in the universe and then relax deeply into the feeling of total 'oneness'.

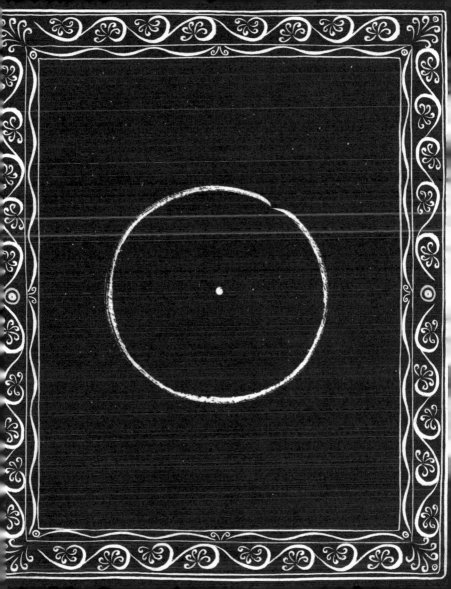

Moving Meditation

There are various forms of 'Moving Meditation' — Martial Arts such as Tai Chi involve a meditative state, and some traditional dance is classed as 'ecstatic' or meditative. Perhaps the best known is the Whirling Dervish, from the mystical branch of Islam called *Sufi*. The Sufi Orders ritualize the *Dhikr* (the Remembrance of God/Allah, involving supplications and repetition of the names of God) through dance and music called the *Sema*. It represents the journey of man's spiritual ascent through mind and love to perfection.

Moving meditation can be what you wish — use it as an expression of your own inner creativity. Breathe rhythmically and deeply, nourish your body and mind. Dance, walk, run or apply it to everyday tasks but keep in mind the object of that which you wish to achieve — be it enlightenment, joy, peace, balance or pure energy!

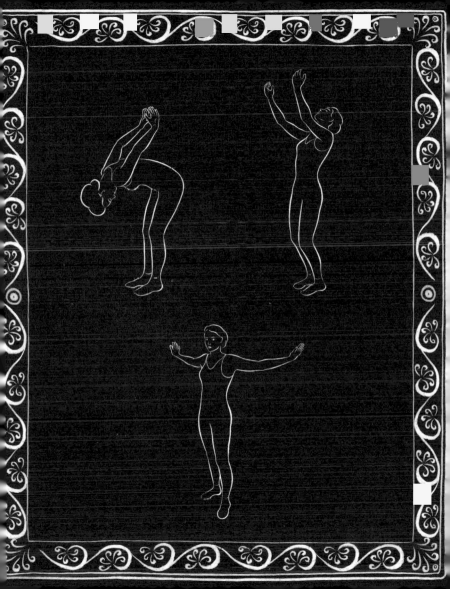

Breathing Meditations

These breathing meditations are taken from the Chinese system of Qigong. *Qi* means air/vitality and *gong* means skill or strength. The three important elements of Qigong are body posture, breathing and mind control — all these you will achieve through meditation. The following exercises are believed to help relax, strengthen and achieve inner growth.

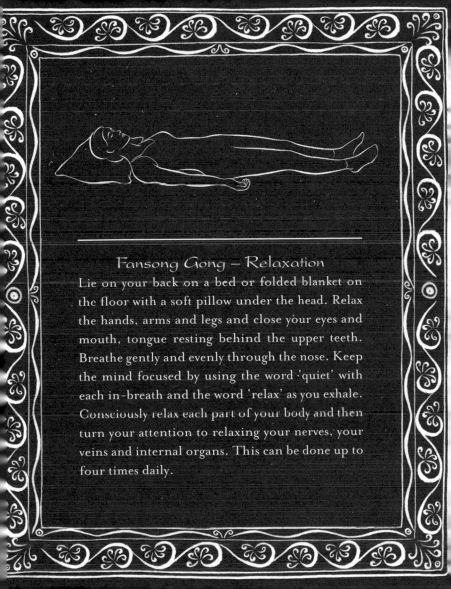

Fansong Gong – Relaxation

Lie on your back on a bed or folded blanket on the floor with a soft pillow under the head. Relax the hands, arms and legs and close your eyes and mouth, tongue resting behind the upper teeth. Breathe gently and evenly through the nose. Keep the mind focused by using the word 'quiet' with each in-breath and the word 'relax' as you exhale. Consciously relax each part of your body and then turn your attention to relaxing your nerves, your veins and internal organs. This can be done up to four times daily.

Qiangzhuang Gong – Strength

Sit erect in Burmese or throne posture, with eyes closed and the tip of your tongue resting behind your upper teeth. Breathe naturally through the nose into your abdomen. Gradually allow your breath to become slower and concentrate on your abdomen by counting 'one' as you inhale, 'two' as you exhale and so on until you reach 'ten' and then repeat. Try to keep your focus on your *Dantien*, the point three inches below your navel, letting any thoughts and distractions flow away.

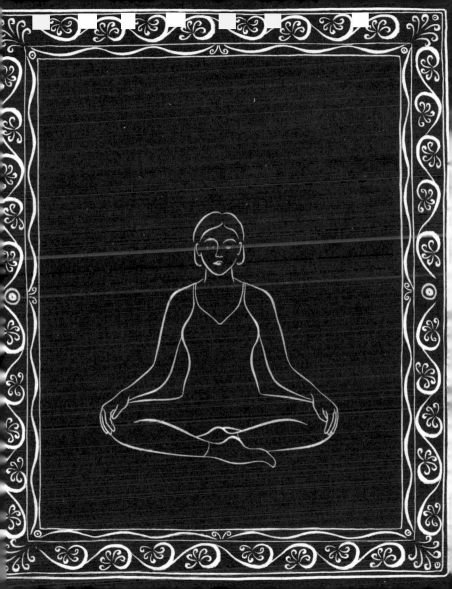

Neiyang Gong – Inner Growth

Neiyang Gong is an exercise of 'change' using auto-suggestion to facilitate inner growth.

This exercise can be done lying or sitting.

Lying on side – Lie on your right side, bending slightly forward with your hand about 2 inches in front of the head, palm up. The left arm rests on hip, palm down. Keep legs bent.

Lying on back – Lie with a pillow under your head, arms at the sides.

Sitting – Sit upright in a chair, feet flat on the ground. Legs separate, shoulder-width apart and hands resting gently on your thighs.

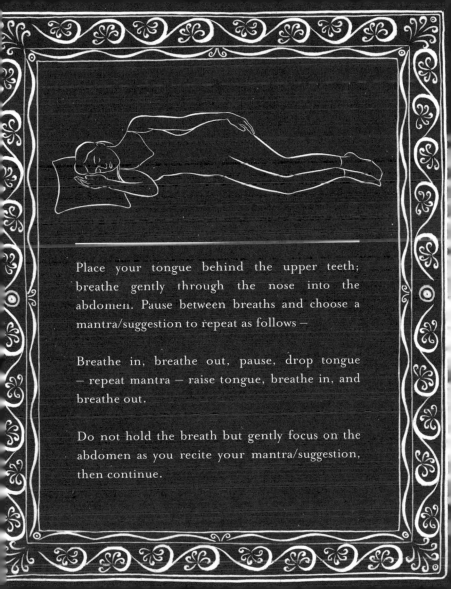

Place your tongue behind the upper teeth; breathe gently through the nose into the abdomen. Pause between breaths and choose a mantra/suggestion to repeat as follows —

Breathe in, breathe out, pause, drop tongue — repeat mantra — raise tongue, breathe in, and breathe out.

Do not hold the breath but gently focus on the abdomen as you recite your mantra/suggestion, then continue.

Meditation for Pregnancy

Meditation during pregnancy is believed to help reduce stress and make the physical process easier to manage. A calm and relaxed mother can contribute to an easier birth and healthier child. The process of deep breathing and focused meditation is a wonderful combination to help mother and child establish an initial bond.

As elaborate seating postures may be difficult, it is safer to adopt a simple Burmese, throne or lying position. Use pillows to make yourself comfortable and to support your back if necessary.

A simple and beautiful meditation to connect with your baby is the following:

Find the most comfortable position for you. Close your eyes and breathe gently and deeply. As you breathe, visualize your child at each stage of its growth surrounded by love and protection.

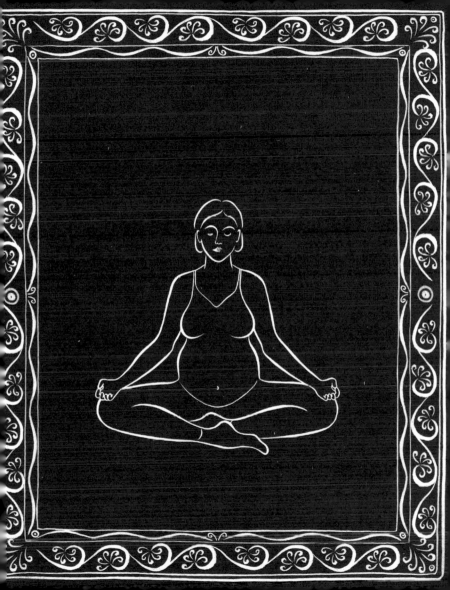

Troubleshooting

As you begin to meditate it is common to experience the following:

- Wandering mind. This is quite natural; just bring yourself back to your point of focus.
- Not sure you are doing it properly? Meditation is pretty simple — just keep practising.
- You have memories or images you have not thought about in years. Acknowledge them and bring your awareness back to your point of focus.
- You start to analyze yourself. This is a time for meditation not psychotherapy.
- You have certain revelations. Again, acknowledge and return to your point of focus.
- A body part is sore or itchy. Acknowledge it and re-focus.